Turning 23: A guide to Healthy Weight Loss (for absolute beginners)

Jesslyn Tan

Contents

Introduction

I've been overweight almost all my life - the last time I was at ideal weight was probably 30 years back.

And just before I turned 40, I decided that I needed to do a few things

> (1) Create a few passive income streams so that I can enjoy life with less financial worries
> (2) Adopt a healthier lifestyle so I can enjoy the life I create

To do (2), I took a long hard look at my health status and lifestyle. While my health has never been too bad, my weight was a disaster zone, with my BMI at 33. Being Asian, this means that I was 10 points above the accepted healthy zone!

I decided to find out how I could get a bit healthier, statistics-wise, and this book records how I lost about 7 kg in 6 months. It would have been more but for 2 birthdays (including mine), Chinese New Year, an epic 12-day Taiwan Trip and the completion of a fairly stressful certification programme.

Understanding the Goal

Getting to the healthier state first requires to know what the healthier state looks like.

For an Asian, the BMI ranges are as follows:

To calculate your BMI, either download any of the free apps or use the formula below:

$$BMI = \frac{Weight\ (Kg)}{(Height\ in\ metres)^2}$$

	BMI range	Target Weight
Underweight	< 18.5	
Optimal Weight	18.5 – 22.9	
Pre-obese	23 – 27.4	
Obese	>27.5	

It helps to record what you started with so you at least know whether what you are doing works for you.

The BMI is however, not the only index you should be looking at. Another key index to look at is the Body Fat index.

There are many ways to do this and I recommend the navy method as you only need an app, weighing scale and tape measure.

Age	BF (Female)	BF (Male)
18 - 21	33	22
22 - 29	34	23
30 - 39	35	24
Over 40	36	26

I also use clothing and bra sizes because I travel to countries where petite sizes are norm (and I really need to buy that dress/top/skirt/bikini). I use cm here.

Bra Size	32	34	36	38
Band Size	68 – 71	73 – 77	78 – 82	83 – 87
A	82 – 84	87 – 89	92 – 94	97 – 99
B	84 – 86	89 – 91	94 – 96	99 – 101
C	86 – 88	91 – 93	96 – 98	101 – 103
D	88 – 90	93 – 95	98 – 100	103 – 105
E/DD	90 – 92	95 – 97	100 – 102	105 – 107
F	92 – 94	97 – 99	102 – 104	107 – 109
G	94 – 96	99 – 101	104 – 106	109 – 111
H	96 – 99	101 - 103	106 - 108	111 – 113

	0	2	4	6	8	10	12	14	16
Bust	84	86	89	91	94	98	102	107	112
Waist	84	66	69	71	74	77	81	86	91
Hip	89	91	94	97	99	103	107	112	117

Now, record your measurements on the last page of this book.

Understanding the Challenges

This next part calls for self-awareness. I'm listing a number of possible reasons why you (and I) are overweight. Circle all that even sound vaguely true.

I eat during times of stress (e.g. when facing a deadline, after an argument)	A		
I (or my family) tend to overcook	A		
I have no time to eat a proper meal and typically have takeaways	A		
I'm too lazy to cook	A		
I hate to sweat		B	
I am too busy to exercise		B	C
I already exercise a lot, so I can eat what I want	A		
I eat when watching TV	A		
I am so overweight I can't exercise		B	
I feel a need to clear all food off the plate	A		
I love all-you-can-eats	A		
I had some recent injuries		B	
I love fast food	A		
I don't even know where to start			C
My typical gatherings with friends and family involve food	A		
I'm too tired to exercise		B	C
It's too expensive to be healthy			C
I can't see results			C
Totals			

Check your results below:

A > 3	Food is necessary for life, and yet, so many of our bad habits are associated with food. We tend to eat during stress and grab whatever food is nearby. At work, we end up eating at our desks as we work through lunch and we tend to do a lot of takeaways to save time. Not to say that takeaways are bad, but we can't see what goes into the cooking! Also, consider exploring a range of activities to do with family and friends that do not involve movies (too much sitting) or eating (for obvious reasons)
B > 2	Most of us do not have sufficient exercise and this can be due to many reasons. We need to educate ourselves on the types of exercise we can do that meets our needs and circumstances and still allow us to stay healthy.
C > 1	You may have the intent to exercise, but have found many reasons not too (too busy, too exercise, too much info). We shall see how we can address that in the coming pages.

For me, it's a mixture of A, B and C.

A:
I am a stress-eater and I really ate mindlessly when I was doing my Masters and Professional Certifications. Being Asians, we are taught from day 1 that wasting of food is a big no-no and yet, mum loves to cook up a storm. I love to bake too and that doesn't quite help. Work can be overwhelming and I eat lunch at my desk several times a week.

B:
Balancing work and school means I had very little free time. Paying my way at school means that I had great motivation to keep my job and yet get the best possible grades in class, which resulted in not even having enough time to sleep, what more time and energy to exercise!

Being very overweight (BMI = 33) and having lighter friends who have knee issues already meant that I was also very cautious not to go down the same route

C:
With the internet being readily available, I had way too many options of 30 day programmes and other challenges to follow. That led to a very confused (and ambitious) planning that led to me giving up after days of exercise!

Understanding the Options

Continuing in the vein of the last chapter, I outline some strategies to deal with each of the possible situations

A:

- I keep healthier snacks around and limit the unhealthy snacks as special treats (limited edition lays and pringles, anyone?)
- I keep a stock of oats and chia seeds at work so that I have a heathier option instead of chicken rice or cup noodles.
- We tried to include brown rice into our daily diet and reduce the number of fast food or takeaway meals
- We limit the amount of sweet drinks in the house

B:

- Being a planner means that I found a need to plan, usually the week in advance. I would plan exercise into my to-do list
- I also researched and classified exercises into 5 levels
- I also remind myself that each day is a fresh start and not overplanning allows me to adjust my plans easily

C:

- Having classified exercises into 5 categories, I started with the easiest and uploaded the rest into google drive! Out of sight, out of mind ☐
- I also bought only what I needed and anything which required massive expenditure was also uploaded for later study
- I used the neighbourhood park and a yoga mat instead of joining a gym
- I also use a weekly tracker for statistics and a daily weight tracker app (just download any from amazon app store or google play)

Tracking Pages

I didn't quite plan for very long term, and you shouldn't too. It's way too tempting to just give up half way because you missed a couple of days (due to work, sickness or an enticing tv programme). Having said that, we should make efforts to be consistent in our exercise.

I'm included the first 3 months of my exercise plans and trackers for absolute beginners to exercising. Turn to the last page of the book and complete the exercises there!

Daily Tracker

It is important to check the type of exercise you get per day! Put a tick in the box if you did the exercise for each day the box isn't greyed out! ☐

	Strength		Cardio		Darebee	
	Plank	Squats	Skip	walk	Challenge	Weight
1						
2						
3						
4						
5						
6						
7						
8						
9						
10						
11						
12						
13						
14						
15						
16						
17						
18						
19						
20						
21						
22						
23						

	Strength		Cardio		Darebee	
24						
25						
	Plank	Squats	Skip	walk	Challenge	Weight
26						
27						
28						
29						
30						
31						
32						
33						
34						
35						
36						
37						
38						
39						
40						
41						
42						
43						
44						
45						
46						
47						
48						
49						
50						
51						
52						
53						
54						
55						
56						
57						

	Strength		Cardio		Darebee	
58						
59						
	Plank	Squats	Skip	walk	Challenge	Weight
60						
61						
62						
63						
64						
65						
66						
67						
68						
69						
70						
71						
72						
73						
74						
75						
76						
77						
78						
79						
80						
81						
82						
83						
84						
85						
86						
87						
88						
89						
90						

Stats Tracker

It is important to measure under similar conditions (I prefer early morning on Sun before breakfast, after washing up)

	Neck	Bust	Band	Waist	Hip
Start Date					
Week 1					
Week 2					
Week 3					
Week 4					
Week 5					
Week 6					
Week 7					
Week 8					
Week 9					
Week 10					
Week 11					
Week 12					
End Date					

	0	2	4	6	8	10	12	14	16
Bust	84	86	89	91	94	98	102	107	112

Waist	84	66	69	71	74	77	81	86	91
Hip	89	91	94	97	99	103	107	112	117

	Weight	Bra Size	Clothes Size	BMI	BF
Start Date					
Week 1					
Week 2					
Week 3					
Week 4					
Week 5					
Week 6					
Week 7					
Week 8					
Week 9					
Week 10					
Week 11					
Week 12					
End Date					

Bra Size	32	34	36	38
Band Size	68 – 71	73 – 77	78 – 82	83 – 87
A	82 – 84	87 – 89	92 – 94	97 – 99
B	84 – 86	89 – 91	94 – 96	99 – 101
C	86 – 88	91 – 93	96 – 98	101 – 103
D	88 – 90	93 – 95	98 – 100	103 – 105
E/DD	90 – 92	95 – 97	100 – 102	105 – 107
F	92 – 94	97 – 99	102 – 104	107 – 109
G	94 – 96	99 – 101	104 – 106	109 – 111
H	96 – 99	101 - 103	106 - 108	111 – 113

Health Diary

I also keep a health diary and I used primarily a few apps and darebee's programmes for my first phase.

Links to items you need to have (in addition to a phone):

Darbee:
Foundation Light
Foundation
Cardio Blast
Totals
Cardio Go

Just 6 weeks

Skipping rope
Skipping programme

Walking Programme

Kickboxing

Note: I've heard of the DVDs being available online. I recommend going legal (they don't cost much). I did and you should too □

Weight Loss Exercise

I rotated through the list of exercises on darebee until I managed to do 1 round at level 3 for all exercises before moving on to the next group. The link is continually updated so do get the list from the website

Group 1 (first 45 days or more)
Link 1 | Link 2

Group 2 (from day 46 or later)
Link 1 | Link 2

While you are at the website, do consider supporting darebee by making a donation!

Day 1

Date:

Day:

Time:

Plank:

Skip:

Challenge: Foundation Light Day 1

Weight:

Day 2

Date:

Day:

Time:

Squats:

Walk:

Challenge: Foundation Light Day 2

Day 3

Date:

Day:

Time:

Plank:

Skip:

Challenge: Foundation Light Day 3

Weight:

Day 4

Date:

Day:

Time:

Squats:

Walk:

Challenge: Foundation Light Day 4

Weight:

Day 5

Date:

Day:

Time:

Plank:

Skip:

Challenge: Foundation Light Day 5

Day 6

Date:

Day:

Time:

Squats:

Walk:

Challenge: Foundation Light Day 6

Weight:

Day 7

Date:

Day:

Time:

Plank:

Skip:

Challenge: Foundation Light Day 7

Day 8

Date:

Day:

Time:

Plank:

Skip:

Challenge: Foundation Light Day 8

Weight:

Day 9

Date:

Day:

Time:

Squats:

Walk:

Challenge: Foundation Light Day 9

Day 10

Date:

Day:

Time:

Plank:

Skip:

Challenge: Foundation Light Day 10

Weight:

Day 11

Date:

Day:

Time:

Squats:

Walk:

Challenge: Foundation Light Day 11

Weight:

Day 12

Date:

Day:

Time:

Plank:

Skip:

Challenge: Foundation Light Day 12

Day 13

Date:

Day:

Time:

Squats:

Walk:

Challenge: Foundation Light Day 13

Weight:

Day 14

Date:

Day:

Time:

Plank:

Skip:

Challenge: Foundation Light Day 14

Day 15

Date:

Day:

Time:

Plank:

Skip:

Challenge: Foundation Light Day 15

Weight:

Day 16

Date:

Day:

Time:

Squats:

Walk:

Challenge: Foundation Light Day 16

Day 17

Date:

Day:

Time:

Plank:

Skip:

Challenge: Foundation Light Day 17

Weight:

Day 18

Date:

Day:

Time:

Squats:

Walk:

Challenge: Foundation Light Day 18

Weight:

Day 19

Date:

Day:

Time:

Plank:

Skip:

Challenge: Foundation Light Day 19

Day 20

Date:

Day:

Time:

Squats:

Walk:

Challenge: Foundation Light Day 20

Weight:

Day 21

Date:

Day:

Time:

Plank:

Skip:

Challenge: Foundation Light Day 21

Day 22

Date:

Day:

Time:

Plank:

Skip:

Challenge: Foundation Light Day 22

Weight:

Day 23

Date:

Day:

Time:

Squats:

Walk:

Challenge: Foundation Light Day 23

Day 24

Date:

Day:

Time:

Plank:

Skip:

Challenge: Foundation Light Day 24

Weight:

Day 25

Date:

Day:

Time:

Squats:

Walk:

Challenge: Foundation Light Day 25

Weight:

Day 26

Date:

Day:

Time:

Plank:

Skip:

Challenge: Foundation Light Day 26

Day 27

Date:

Day:

Time:

Squats:

Walk:

Challenge: Foundation Light Day 27

Weight:

Day 28

Date:

Day:

Time:

Plank:

Skip:

Challenge: Foundation Light Day 28

Day 29

Date:

Day:

Time:

Plank:

Skip:

Challenge: Foundation Light Day 29

Weight:

Day 30

Date:

Day:

Time:

Squats:

Walk:

Challenge: Foundation Light Day 30

Day 31

Date:

Day:

Time:

Plank:

Skip:

Challenge: **Foundation** / **Cardio Blast** Day 1

Weight:

Day 32

Date:

Day:

Time:

Squats:

Walk:

Challenge: **Foundation** / **Cardio Blast** Day 2

Weight:

Day 33

Date:

Day:

Time:

Plank:

Skip:

Challenge: Foundation / Cardio Blast Day 3

Day 34

Date:

Day:

Time:

Squats:

Walk:

Challenge: Foundation / Cardio Blast Day 4

Weight:

Day 35

Date:

Day:

Time:

Plank:

Skip:

Challenge: Foundation / Cardio Blast Day 5

Day 36

Date:

Day:

Time:

Plank:

Skip:

Challenge: Foundation / Cardio Blast Day 6

Weight:

Day 37

Date:

Day:

Time:

Squats:

Walk:

Challenge: Foundation / Cardio Blast Day 7

Day 38

Date:

Day:

Time:

Plank:

Skip:

Challenge: Foundation / Cardio Blast Day 8

Weight:

Day 39

Date:

Day:

Time:

Squats:

Walk:

Challenge: Foundation / Cardio Blast Day 9

Weight:

Day 40

Date:

Day:

Time:

Plank:

Skip:

Challenge: Foundation / Cardio Blast Day 10

Day 41

Date:

Day:

Time:

Squats:

Walk:

Challenge: Foundation / Cardio Blast Day 11

Weight:

Day 42

Date:

Day:

Time:

Plank:

Skip:

Challenge: Foundation / Cardio Blast Day 12

Day 43

Date:

Day:

Time:

Plank:

Skip:

Challenge: Foundation / Cardio Blast Day 13

Weight:

Day 44

Date:

Day:

Time:

Squats:

Walk:

Challenge: Foundation / Cardio Blast Day 14

Day 45

Date:

Day:

Time:

Plank:

Skip:

Challenge: Foundation / Cardio Blast Day 15

Weight:

Day 46

Date:

Day:

Time:

Squats:

Walk:

Challenge: Foundation / Cardio Blast Day 16

Weight:

Day 47

Date:

Day:

Time:

Plank:

Skip:

Challenge: Foundation / Cardio Blast Day 17

Day 48

Date:

Day:

Time:

Squats:

Walk:

Challenge: Foundation / Cardio Blast Day 18

Weight:

Day 49

Date:

Day:

Time:

Plank:

Skip:

Challenge: Foundation / Cardio Blast Day 19

Day 50

Date:

Day:

Time:

Plank:

Skip:

Challenge: Foundation / Cardio Blast Day 20

Weight:

Day 51

Date:

Day:

Time:

Squats:

Walk:

Challenge: Foundation / Cardio Blast Day 21

Day 52

Date:

Day:

Time:

Plank:

Skip:

Challenge: Foundation / Cardio Blast Day 22

Weight:

Day 53

Date:

Day:

Time:

Squats:

Walk:

Challenge: Foundation / Cardio Blast Day 23

Weight:

Day 54

Date:

Day:

Time:

Plank:

Skip:

Challenge: Foundation / Cardio Blast Day 24

Day 55

Date:

Day:

Time:

Squats:

Walk:

Challenge: Foundation / Cardio Blast Day 25

Weight:

Day 56

Date:

Day:

Time:

Plank:

Skip:

Challenge: Foundation / Cardio Blast Day 26

Day 57

Date:

Day:

Time:

Plank:

Skip:

Challenge: Foundation / Cardio Blast Day 27

Weight:

Day 58

Date:

Day:

Time:

Squats:

Walk:

Challenge: Foundation / Cardio Blast Day 28

Day 59

Date:

Day:

Time:

Plank:

Skip:

Challenge: Foundation / Cardio Blast Day 29

Weight:

Day 60

Date:

Day:

Time:

Squats:

Walk:

Challenge: Foundation / Cardio Blast Day 30

Weight:

Day 61

Date:

Day:

Time:

Plank:

Skip:

Challenge: Totals / Cardio Go Day 1

Day 62

Date:

Day:

Time:

Squats:

Walk:

Challenge: Totals / Cardio Go Day 2

Weight:

Day 63

Date:

Day:

Time:

Plank:

Skip:

Challenge: Totals / Cardio Go Day 3

Day 64

Date:

Day:

Time:

Plank:

Skip:

Challenge: Totals / Cardio Go Day 4

Weight:

Day 65

Date:

Day:

Time:

Squats:

Walk:

Challenge: Totals / Cardio Go Day 5

Day 66

Date:

Day:

Time:

Plank:

Skip:

Challenge: Totals / Cardio Go Day 6

Weight:

Day 67

Date:

Day:

Time:

Squats:

Walk:

Challenge: Totals / Cardio Go Day 7

Weight:

Day 68

Date:

Day:

Time:

Plank:

Skip:

Challenge: Totals / Cardio Go Day 8

Day 69

Date:

Day:

Time:

Squats:

Walk:

Challenge: Totals / Cardio Go Day 9

Weight:

Day 70

Date:

Day:

Time:

Plank:

Skip:

Challenge: Totals / Cardio Go Day 10

Day 71

Date:

Day:

Time:

Plank:

Skip:

Challenge: Totals / Cardio Go Day 11

Weight:

Day 72

Date:

Day:

Time:

Squats:

Walk:

Challenge: Totals / Cardio Go Day 12

Day 73

Date:

Day:

Time:

Plank:

Skip:

Challenge: Totals / Cardio Go Day 13

Weight:

Day 74

Date:

Day:

Time:

Squats:

Walk:

Challenge: Totals / Cardio Go Day 14

Weight:

Day 75

Date:

Day:

Time:

Plank:

Skip:

Challenge: Totals / Cardio Go Day 15

Day 76

Date:

Day:

Time:

Squats:

Walk:

Challenge: Totals / Cardio Go Day 16

Weight:

Day 77

Date:

Day:

Time:

Plank:

Skip:

Challenge: Totals / Cardio Go Day 17

Day 78

Date:

Day:

Time:

Plank:

Skip:

Challenge: Totals / Cardio Go Day 18

Weight:

Day 79

Date:

Day:

Time:

Squats:

Walk:

Challenge: Totals / Cardio Go Day 19

Day 80

Date:

Day:

Time:

Plank:

Skip:

Challenge: Totals / Cardio Go Day 20

Weight:

Day 81

Date:

Day:

Time:

Squats:

Walk:

Challenge: Totals / Cardio Go Day 21

Weight:

Day 82

Date:

Day:

Time:

Plank:

Skip:

Challenge: Totals / Cardio Go Day 22

Day 83

Date:

Day:

Time:

Squats:

Walk:

Challenge: Totals / Cardio Go Day 23

Weight:

Day 84

Date:

Day:

Time:

Plank:

Skip:

Challenge: Totals / Cardio Go Day 24

Day 85

Date:

Day:

Time:

Plank:

Skip:

Challenge: Totals / Cardio Go Day 25

Weight:

Day 86

Date:

Day:

Time:

Squats:

Walk:

Challenge: Totals / Cardio Go Day 26

Day 87

Date:

Day:

Time:

Plank:

Skip:

Challenge: Totals / Cardio Go Day 27

Weight:

Day 88

Date:

Day:

Time:

Squats:

Walk:

Challenge: Totals / Cardio Go Day 28

Weight:

Day 89

Date:

Day:

Time:

Plank:

Skip:

Challenge: Totals / Cardio Go Day 29

Day 90

Date:

Day:

Time:

Squats:

Walk:

Challenge: Totals / Cardio Go Day 30

Weight:

Frequently Asked Questions

1. What happens if I miss a day (or more)?

   This happens to the best of us. Simply carry on with the next day and take care not to over exert. If you need to, stop when you have reached your maximum and repeat that level (instead of progressing to the next)

2. When will I see the effects of exercising?

   It is said that you will see the effects after 2 weeks, your loved ones after 4 and others after 8. I saw decreases in weight and stats after a few days although visually, we couldn't tell (partly because of the clothes, perhaps?)

3. I nearly died today while doing this level. What should I do?

You should repeat each level until you feel comfortable with it. You know your own body best – and you should be progressing at your own pace!

Before and After

	Day 1	Day 90
Date:		
Using your tape measure		
Neck		
Bust		
Band size		
Waist		
Hip		
Using your weighing scale		
Weight		
Using apps or calculator		
BMI		
Body Fat		
Using the tables in this chapter		
Bra		
Dress		
Exercises		
Duration of plank		
No of Squats		
Distance walked without panting[1]		

---

[1] Aim for a pace of 15 min per 1.6km